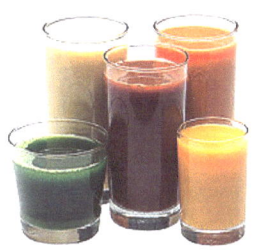

Healing Juicing, Smoothie and Milk Shake Recipes

Juices Smoothies, and Milk Shakes that Help the Body Achieve its Self-Healing Process

Adetutu Ijose

JP

Copyright © 2009

Jointheirs Publishing
Jointheirs Activities Incorporated
www.jointheirspublishing.com

ISBN -: 1-44951-553-3

EAN – 978-1-44951-553-9.

Printed in the United States of America

Dedication

This book is dedicated to God my Creator who through his Spirit gave me the recipes that are in this book when I had life threatening health issues and man made systems could not help. To him alone be the glory for this book.

Healing Juicing, Smoothie and Milk Shake Recipes

Juices Smoothies, and Milk Shakes that help the Body Achieve its self-healing process

Acknowledgements

Many individuals have contributed to the completion of this book. I wish to acknowledge all who have encouraged me to write more books and provide help to others with the knowledge God has given me so that they can receive their healing as I have received mine. Thanks to all.

An Important Caution

These recipes are based on personal experience. It is important that you discuss any dietary change or choices you make with your doctor before adopting any recipe to ensure that is nothing in the ingredients that can interfere with your medication or anything else being provided to you. These recipes do not replace the advise of your nutritionist or doctor who know you well. Again please discuss these recipes with them before starting. Also remember individual results will vary and that the individual way you follow these recipes e.g. the quality of the ingredients, juicing method etc. Could affect the result

Table of Content

Preface

This book is intended to be a health and nutrition guide for anyone looking for way of boosting their general health, immune system function and body cleanse naturally. The juices will provide cleansing. I take my juice daily as the last thing about an hour or two after my dinner. The smoothies and shakes could be taken in between meals instead of snacks. You can freeze them and take a glassful to work everyday and take it to boost your energy during the day.

Chapter I
Introduction

The body depends on nutrients from the foods we eat to replenish itself and to provide the energy for our daily activities as well as to carry out tissue and cell repair and defence. Today's environment is full of chemicals and pollutants from industrialization and our technology dependent way of life. These chemical and pollutants are harmful to our bodies that therefore need more resources to keep us healthy than in previous generations where there was not as much pollution.

Sadly however, our soils are polluted and depleted and consequently the foods we have are not as healthy as those in previous years. Added to this pollution are the chemicals from pesticides and herbicides we use to ensure a more bountiful harvest. Further we have genetically modified and engineered the seeds that we no longer really know what we are eating.

Many of today's sicknesses and disease are a direct result of all the above making it very important to do the best we can to ensure we eat healthily. If you are suffering any kind of health condition these recipes will truly assist in the healing process.
Okay enough said. Now go ahead enjoy your juice. I encourage you to make juicing a daily event. If you do, you will begin to notice a difference in your health.

Note for All

You may take your juice in the morning or in the evening as the last thing you take. That is what I do. I take my juice in the evening. I find it most beneficial then as it helps in digesting my diner. Remember diet must be complemented by a good exercise routine including walking and other outdoor exercises. Apart from juices, smoothies and milk shakes, I find that taking an orange or grapefruit after every meal helps to digest the meal and assists with the elimination of waste as these citrus fruits contain a lot of fiber when everything is eaten i.e. the core, seed and white inner peel. Just take off the skin and eat the rest. Consequently a juicer that includes the pulp in the juice is I believe healthier.

If you have any particular health conditions or are on some medication, I will advise consulting with your doctor about your food to ensure that nothing in the foods you eat interacts with your medication preventing them from bcing effective or that makes them counter productive.

Juices, Smoothies and Milk Shakes

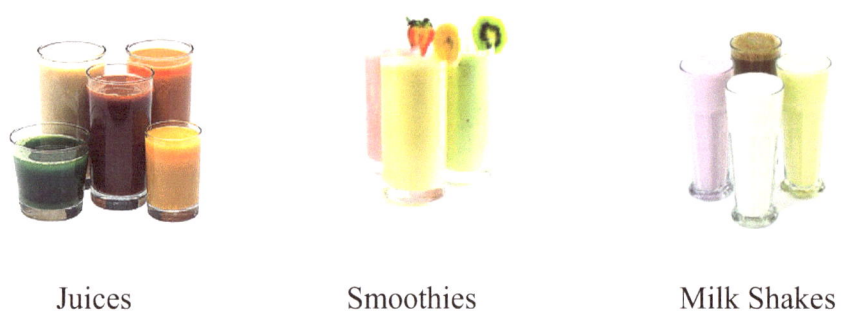

Juices   Smoothies   Milk Shakes

Fruits and Vegetables are important building blocks for a health life style. Many a times they become boring especially for children. In addition some are sweeter than others and in fact some vegetables are near bitter or bitter. To ensure that we get the essential nutrients we need it is important to make them all interesting and sweet. The easiest way to do this is to juice them, or make them into smoothies or milk shakes.

There is a temptation to believe that we can avoid taking fruits and vegetables by taking supplements. Our bodies were however not made for supplements but for obtaining nutrients by processing the food we eat. Consequently our bodies do not absorb all the nutrients in the supplements we take. Further some supplements are not from natural sources and may leave residues in our systems that our bodies were not designed with the capacity to break down and that therefore create their own problems in our bodies.

In fact the reason they are called supplements is because they are not designed to be substitutes but supplements when we are unable to get enough of the natural forms into our system due to illnesses or our bodies inability to process certain food components, or allergies or inadequate supplies in the foods themselves (due to the depletion of the soil in which they are grown).

.

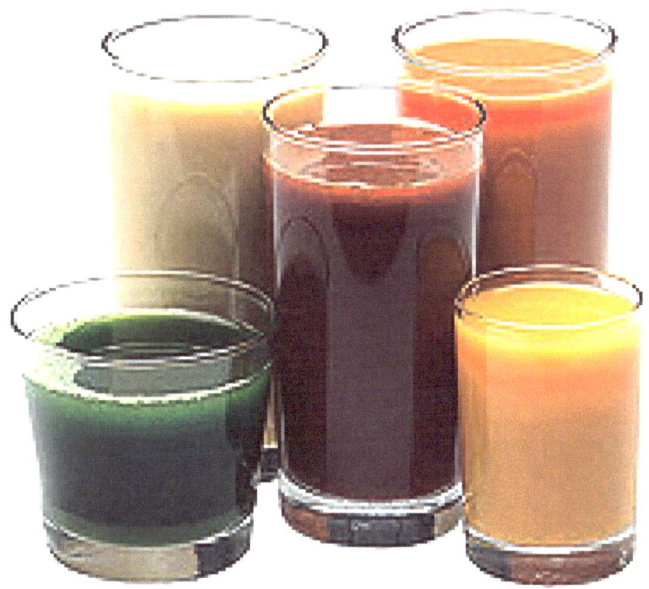

Chapter II
Fruit/Vegetable Juicing

Juicing breaks down the food items into a state that makes it easier for the body to absorb the nutrients in them. If you do not have or are unable to obtain any of the ingredients in the recipe just use what you have and substitute with other suitable ones available to you.

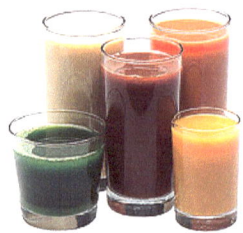

Sweet Citrus and Vegetable Juice

It is healthier to use organic ingredients to avoid chemicals and pesticides that add excesses estrogens and harmful chemicals. Conventional fruits and vegetables are heavily sprayed.

Ingredients

1 Organic Orange
1 Small Organic Grapefruit
1 Organic Lemon
1 Organic (if possible. I buy mine from Shoprite) Mango
I Organic Peach
1/4 Cup of Organic Cauliflower
1/2 Stick if Organic Celery including the leaf if available
1 Small Organic Collard Green leaf
½ -1 Organic Kale leaf
A Piece of Ginger about the size of an orange seed.

Remove only the skin from the Orange, lemon and grapefruit but leave the white peel and the seeds. The peel and seeds are very nutritional. Cut all the fruits and vegetable into small pieces. Either juice everything together using a juicer if you have one or else blend all in a blender. You may want to add water if you find it too concentrated.

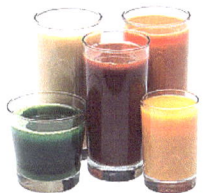

Sweet Citrus, Berries and vegetable Juice

It is healthier to use organic ingredients to avoid chemicals and pesticides that add excesses estrogens and harmful chemicals. Conventional fruits and vegetables are heavily sprayed.

Ingredients

1 Organic Orange
1 Small Organic Grapefruit
1 Organic Lemon
Organic Strawberries
Organic Raspberries
Organic blueberries
1/2 Stick if Organic Celery (including the leaf if available)
1 Small Organic Collard Green leaf
A Piece of Ginger about the size of an orange seed.

Remove only the skin from the Orange, lemon and grapefruit but leave the white peel and the seeds. The peel and seeds are very nutritional. Cut all the fruits and vegetable into small pieces. Either juice everything together using a juicer if you have one or else blend all in a blender. You may want to add water if you find it too concentrated.

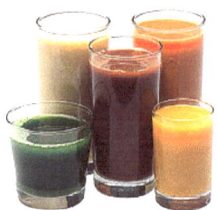

Sweet Citrus, Banana and Vegetable Juice

It is healthier to use organic ingredients to avoid chemicals and pesticides that add excesses estrogens and harmful chemicals. Conventional fruits and vegetables are heavily sprayed.

Ingredients

1 Organic Orange
1 Small Organic Grapefruit
1 Organic Lemon
1 Organic (if possible. I buy mine from Shoprite) Mango
1 Organic Apple
1 Organic Banana
1/2 Stick if Organic Celery (including the leaf if available)
Organic beet leaves
A Piece of Ginger about the size of an orange seed.

Remove only the skin from the Orange, lemon and grapefruit but leave the white peel and the seeds. The peel and seeds are very nutritional. Cut all the fruits and vegetable into small pieces. Either juice everything together using a juicer if you have one or else blend all in a blender. You may want to add water if you find it too concentrated.

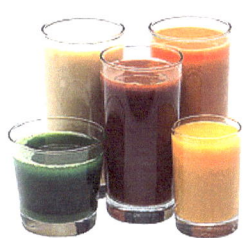

Sweet Citrus Carrots and Green Vegetable Juice

It is healthier to use organic ingredients to avoid chemicals and pesticides that add excesses estrogens and harmful chemicals. Conventional fruits and vegetables are heavily sprayed.

Ingredients

1 Organic Orange
1 Small Organic Grapefruit
1 Organic Lemon
1 Organic (if possible.) Mango
I Organic Peach
1 Organic Sweet Nectarine
Organic Carrots
1/2 Stick if Organic Celery (including the leaf if available)
1 Small Organic Collard Green leaf
½ -1 Organic Kale leaf
A Piece of Ginger about the size of an orange seed.

Remove only the skin from the Orange, lemon and grapefruit but leave the white peel and the seeds. The peel and seeds are very nutritional. Cut all the fruits and vegetable into small pieces. Either juice everything together using a juicer if you have one or else blend all in a blender. You may want to add water if you find it too concentrated.

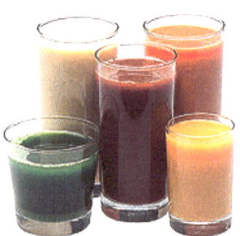

Lemon, pineapple Carrots and Green Vegetable Juice

It is healthier to use organic ingredients to avoid chemicals and pesticides that add excesses estrogens and harmful chemicals. Conventional fruits and vegetables are heavily sprayed.

Ingredients

1 Organic Orange
1 Small Pineapple
1 Organic Lemon
1 Organic (if possible. I buy mine from Shoprite) Mango
1 Organic Sweet peach
Organic Carrots
1/2 Stick if Organic Celery (including the leaf if available) - optional
1 Organic beet or small collard green leaf
½ -1 Organic Kale leaf
A Piece of Ginger about the size of an orange seed.

Remove only the skin from the Orange, lemon and grapefruit but leave the white peel and the seeds. The peel and seeds are very nutritional. Cut all the fruits and vegetable into small pieces. Either juice everything together using a juicer if you have one or else blend all in a blender. You may want to add water if you find it too concentrated.

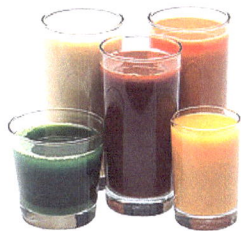

Sweet Citrus Papaya, Pineapple, Apple and Vegetable Juice

It is healthier to use organic ingredients to avoid chemicals and pesticides that add excesses estrogens and harmful chemicals. Conventional fruits and vegetables are heavily sprayed.

Ingredients

1 Organic Orange
1 Small Papaya
1 Small Pineapple
1 Organic Lemon
1 Organic (if possible. I buy mine from Shoprite) Mango
I Organic Apple
1 Organic Tomato
1/2 Stick if Organic Celery (including the leaf if available)
1 Small Organic Collard Green leaf or some Spinach
½ -1 Organic Kale leaf (optional)
A Piece of Ginger about the size of an orange seed.

Remove only the skin from the Orange, and lemon but leave the white peel and the seeds. The peel and seeds are very nutritional. Cut all the fruits and vegetable into small pieces. Either juice everything together using a juicer if you have one or else blend all in a blender. You may want to add water if you find it too concentrated.

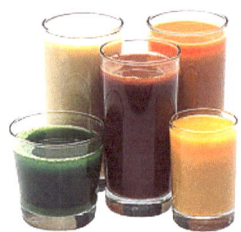

Sweet Cantaloupe, Lemon, Orange and Vegetable Juice

It is healthier to use organic ingredients to avoid chemicals and pesticides that add excesses estrogens and harmful chemicals. Conventional fruits and vegetables are heavily sprayed.

Ingredients

1 Organic Orange
1 Small Cantaloupe (Organic if possible)
1 Organic Lemon
1/4 Cup of Organic Cauliflower
1/2 Stick if Organic Celery (including the leaf if available)
1 Small Organic Collard Green leaf or some Spinach
½ -1 Organic Kale leaf (optional)
A Piece of Ginger about the size of an orange seed.

Remove only the skin from the Orange, and lemon but leave the white peel and the seeds. The peel and seeds are very nutritional. Cut all the fruits and vegetable into small pieces. Either juice everything together using a juicer if you have one or else blend all in a blender. You may want to add water if you find it too concentrated.

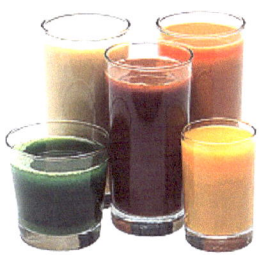

Sweet Melon Lemon, Orange and Vegetable Juice

It is healthier to use organic ingredients to avoid chemicals and pesticides that add excesses estrogens and harmful chemicals. Conventional fruits and vegetables are heavily sprayed.

Ingredients

1 Organic Orange
1 Small Melon (Organic if possible)
1 Small Pineapple
1 Organic Lemon
1/2 Cup of Organic Cauliflower
1/2 Stick if Organic Celery (including the leaf if available)
1 Small Organic Collard Green leaf or some Spinach
½ -1 Organic Kale leaf (optional)
A Piece of Ginger about the size of an orange seed.

Remove only the skin from the Orange, and lemon but leave the white peel and the seeds. The peel and seeds are very nutritional. Cut all the fruits and vegetable into small pieces. Either juice everything together using a juicer if you have one or else blend all in a blender. You may want to add water if you find it too concentrated.

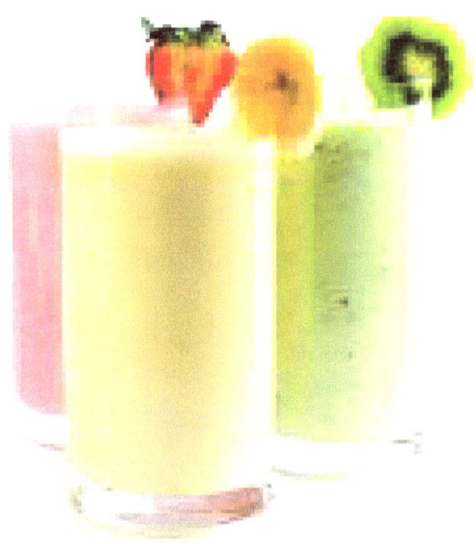

Chapter III
Healing Smoothies

These recipes in some cases non-milk and in some case use almond, rice or skim/non-fat cow milk. You can substitute them for each other if you are unable to obtain the one required for a particular recipe. If you do not have or are unable to obtain any of the other ingredients in the recipe just use what you have and substitute with other suitable ones available to you.

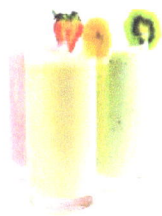

Sweet Citrus and Almond Milk Smoothie

It is healthier to use organic ingredients to avoid chemicals and pesticides that add excesses estrogens and harmful chemicals. Conventional fruits and vegetables are heavily sprayed.

Ingredients – You may freeze the fruits and vegetables pieces first or buy the frozen version for a thicker smoothie.

1 Organic Orange
1 Small Organic Grapefruit
1 Organic Lemon
1 Organic (if possible.) Mango
1 Organic Banana
½ Cup of Shredded Almonds (Organic if possible) you can buy the whole almonds and cut them up yourself
Organic plain non-fat/Skim Yogurt (if possible use organic grass fed cow milk yogurt)
½ to 1 Cup of Organic Almond Milk
Ice cubes

Remove only the skin from the Orange, lemon and grapefruit but leave the white peel and the seeds. The peel and seeds are very nutritional. Cut all the fruits and vegetable into small pieces. Blend everything together with the almonds, yogurt and almond milk and ice cubes in a blender. Scoop it all out into glass cups and serve.

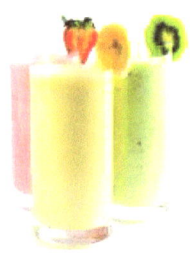

Sweet Citrus and Almond Nuts Smoothie

It is healthier to use organic ingredients to avoid chemicals and pesticides that add excesses estrogens and harmful chemicals. Conventional fruits and vegetables are heavily sprayed.

Ingredients – You may freeze the fruits and vegetables pieces first or buy the frozen version for a thicker smoothie.

1 Organic Orange
1 Small Organic Grapefruit
1 Organic Lemon
1 Organic (if possible.) Mango
1 Organic Banana
½ Cup of Shredded almonds (Organic if possible) you can buy the whole almonds and cut them up yourself
Ice cubes

Remove only the skin from the Orange, lemon and grapefruit but leave the white peel and the seeds. The peel and seeds are very nutritional. Cut all the fruits and vegetable into small pieces. Blend everything together with the almonds and ice cubes in a blender. Scoop it all out into glass cups and serve.

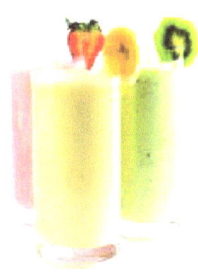

Sweet Citrus and Carrots Smoothie

It is healthier to use organic ingredients to avoid chemicals and pesticides that add excesses estrogens and harmful chemicals. Conventional fruits and vegetables are heavily sprayed.

Ingredients – You may freeze the fruits and vegetables pieces first or buy the frozen version for a thicker smoothie.

1 Organic Orange
1 Small Organic Grapefruit
1 Organic Lemon
1 Organic (if possible.) Mango
1 Cup of Organic Carrots
½ to 1 Cup of Organic (if possible organic grass fed) Milk
A Piece of Ginger about the size of an orange seed.
Ice cubes

Remove only the skin from the Orange, lemon and grapefruit but leave the white peel and the seeds. The peel and seeds are very nutritional. Cut all the fruits and vegetable into small pieces. Blend everything together with the ice cubes in a blender. Scoop it all out into glass cups and serve.

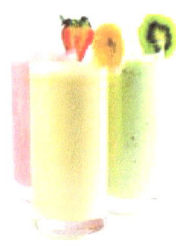

Sweet Citrus, Banana and Vegetable Smoothie

It is healthier to use organic ingredients to avoid chemicals and pesticides that add excesses estrogens and harmful chemicals. Conventional fruits and vegetables are heavily sprayed.

Ingredients – You may freeze the fruits and vegetables pieces first or buy the frozen version for a thicker smoothie..

1 Organic Orange
1 Small Organic Grapefruit
1 Organic Lemon
1 Organic (if possible.) Mango
I Organic Banana
I small stick of Organic Celery
I1/2 Organic Kale leaf
A Piece of Ginger about the size of an orange seed.
½ to 1 Cup of Organic (if possible organic grass fed) skim or non fat Milk
1 Teaspoon of Organic Honey (optional)
Ice cubes

Remove only the skin from the Orange, lemon and grapefruit but leave the white peel and the seeds. The peel and seeds are very nutritional. Cut all the fruits and vegetable into small pieces. Blend everything together with the milk and ice cubes in a blender. Scoop it all out into glass cups and serve..

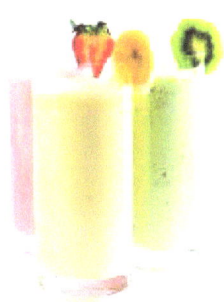

Sweet Citrus, Carrots and Molasses Smoothie

It is healthier to use organic ingredients to avoid chemicals and pesticides that add excesses estrogens and harmful chemicals. Conventional fruits and vegetables are heavily sprayed.

Ingredients – You may freeze the fruits and vegetables pieces first or buy the frozen version for a thicker smoothie..

1 Organic Orange
1 Small Organic Grapefruit
1 Organic Lemon
1 Organic (if possible.) Mango
1 cup of Organic Carrots
1 Teaspoon of Organic Molasses
Ice cubes

Remove only the skin from the Orange, lemon and grapefruit but leave the white peel and the seeds. The peel and seeds are very nutritional. Cut all the fruits and vegetable into small pieces. Blend everything together with the molasses and ice cubes in a blender. Scoop it all out into glass cups and serve.

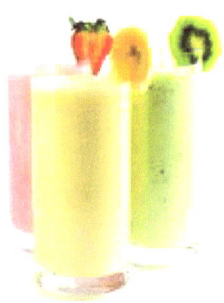

Mixed Berries, Carrots and Brown Rice Smoothie

It is healthier to use organic ingredients to avoid chemicals and pesticides that add excesses estrogens and harmful chemicals. Conventional fruits and vegetables are heavily sprayed.

Ingredients – You may freeze the fruits and vegetables pieces first or buy the frozen version for a thicker smoothie..

1 Cup of Organic Strawberries
1 Cup of Organic Raspberries
1 Cup of Organic Blueberries
I Cup of Organic Brown Rice
1 Cup of Organic Carrots
½ to 1 Cup of Organic Rice Milk
Ice cubes

Remove only the skin from the Orange, lemon and grapefruit but leave the white peel and the seeds. The peel and seeds are very nutritional. Cut all the fruits and vegetable into small pieces. Blend everything together with the brown rice, ice cubes and rice milk in a blender. Scoop it all out into glass cups and serve.

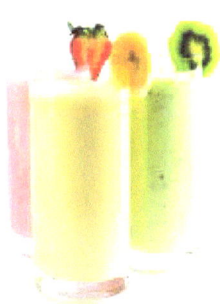

Peaches and Banana Smoothie

It is healthier to use organic ingredients to avoid chemicals and pesticides that add excesses estrogens and harmful chemicals. Conventional fruits and vegetables are heavily sprayed.

Ingredients – You may freeze the fruits and vegetables pieces first or buy the frozen version for a thicker smoothie.

I to 2 Organic Peaches
1 Organic Banana
1 Tablespoonful of Organic plain Yogurt
½ to 1 Cup of Organic (if possible organic grass fed) Milk
Ice cubes

Remove only the skin from the Orange, lemon and grapefruit but leave the white peel and the seeds. The peel and seeds are very nutritional. Cut all the fruits and vegetable into small pieces. Either juice everything together using a juicer if you have one or else blend all in a blender. You may want to add water if you find it too concentrated.

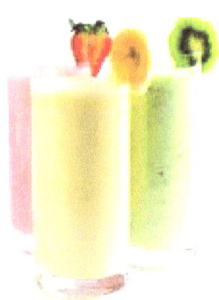

Sweet Nectarines, Banana and Organic Celery Honey Smoothie

It is healthier to use organic ingredients to avoid chemicals and pesticides that add excesses estrogens and harmful chemicals. Conventional fruits and vegetables are heavily sprayed.

Ingredients – You may freeze the fruits and vegetables pieces first or buy the frozen version for a thicker smoothie.

3 Organic Sweet Nectarines
1 Organic Banana
1 Stick if Organic Celery (including the leaf if available)
1 Tablespoons of Organic Plain Yogurt
½ Teaspoon of Organic Honey
Ice cubes

Remove only the skin from the Orange, lemon and grapefruit but leave the white peel and the seeds. The peel and seeds are very nutritional. Cut all the fruits and vegetable into small pieces. Blend everything together with the ice cubes in a blender. Scoop it all out into glass cups and serve.

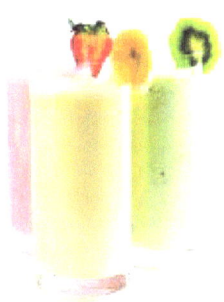

Banana, Carrots and Almond Smoothie

It is healthier to use organic ingredients to avoid chemicals and pesticides that add excesses estrogens and harmful chemicals. Conventional fruits and vegetables are heavily sprayed.

Ingredients – You may freeze the fruits and vegetables pieces first or buy the frozen version for a thicker smoothie.

3 Organic Banana
1 cup Organic Carrots
½ Cup of Shredded Almonds (Organic if possible) you can buy the whole almonds and cut them up yourself
A Piece of Ginger about the size of an orange seed.
Ice cubes

Remove only the skin from the Orange, lemon and grapefruit but leave the white peel and the seeds. The peel and seeds are very nutritional. Cut all the banana and carrots into small pieces. Blend everything together with the ice cubes and ginger in a blender. Scoop it all out into glass cups and serve.

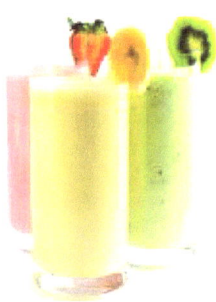

Sweet Green Vegetable and Almond Smoothie

It is healthier to use organic ingredients to avoid chemicals and pesticides that add excesses estrogens and harmful chemicals. Conventional fruits and vegetables are heavily sprayed.

Ingredients – You may freeze the fruits and vegetables pieces first or buy the frozen version for a thicker smoothie.

1 Organic Swiss Chard Leaf
1 Organic Beet Leaf
1 Stick if Organic Celery (including the leaf if available)
1 Organic Collard Green leaf
1 Organic Kale leaf
1 Tablespoonful of shredded Almonds (Organic if possible).. You can also use regular almonds
A Piece of Ginger about the size of an orange seed.
1 tablespoon of Organic honey
Ice cubes

Remove only the skin from the Orange, lemon and grapefruit but leave the white peel and the seeds. The peel and seeds are very nutritional. Cut all the banana and carrots into small pieces. Blend everything together with the almonds, honey, ice cubes and ginger in a blender. Scoop it all out into glass cups and serve.

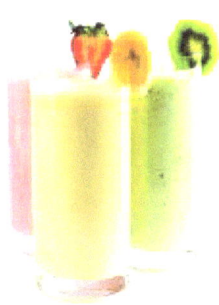

Sweet Citrus Green Vegetable and Carrots Smoothie

It is healthier to use organic ingredients to avoid chemicals and pesticides that add excesses estrogens and harmful chemicals. Conventional fruits and vegetables are heavily sprayed.

Ingredients – You may freeze the fruits and vegetables pieces first or buy the frozen version for a thicker smoothie.

1 Organic Orange
1 Organic (if possible.) Mango
Organic Carrots
1/2 Stick if Organic Celery (including the leaf if available)
1 Small Organic Collard Green leaf
½ -1 Organic Kale leaf
A Piece of Ginger about the size of an orange seed.
Ice cubes

Remove only the skin from the Orange, lemon and grapefruit but leave the white peel and the seeds. The peel and seeds are very nutritional. Cut all the banana and carrots into small pieces. Blend everything together with the ice cubes and ginger in a blender. Scoop it all out into glass cups and serve.

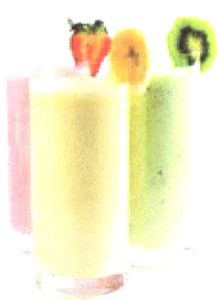

Sweet Green Vegetable and Banana Smoothie

It is healthier to use organic ingredients to avoid chemicals and pesticides that add excesses estrogens and harmful chemicals. Conventional fruits and vegetables are heavily sprayed.

Ingredients – You may freeze the fruits and vegetables pieces first or buy the frozen version for a thicker smoothie.

1 Organic Banana
1/2 Stick if Organic Celery (including the leaf if available)
1 Small Organic Collard Green leaf
½ -1 Organic Kale leaf
½ Cup of plain or Organic Banana Yogurt (if possible get organic grass fed cow yogurt)
1 spoonful of Organic Molasses
A Piece of Ginger about the size of an orange seed.
Ice Cubes

Remove only the skin from the Orange, lemon and grapefruit but leave the white peel and the seeds. The peel and seeds are very nutritional. Cut all the banana and carrots into small pieces. Blend everything together with the molasses, yogurt, ice cubes and ginger in a blender. Scoop it all out into glass cups and serve.

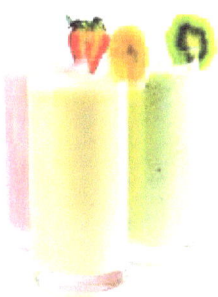

Sweet Green Vegetable and Cantaloupe Smoothie

It is healthier to use organic ingredients to avoid chemicals and pesticides that add excesses estrogens and harmful chemicals. Conventional fruits and vegetables are heavily sprayed.

Ingredients – You may freeze the fruits and vegetables pieces first or buy the frozen version for a thicker smoothie.

1 Organic (if possible) Cantaloupe
1/2 Stick if Organic Celery (including the leaf if available)
1 Small Organic Collard Green leaf
½ -1 Organic Kale leaf
1 Organic Swiss Chard or Beer Leaf
1 Teaspoonful of Organic Honey
Ice Cubes

Peel the cantaloupe. Cut all the vegetables and cantaloupe into small pieces. Blend everything together with the honey, ice cubes and ginger in a blender. Scoop it all out into glass cups and serve.

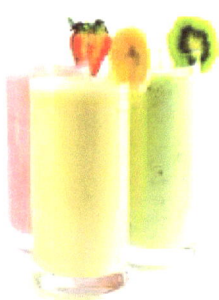

Sweet Green Vegetable Peaches and Mango Smoothie

It is healthier to use organic ingredients to avoid chemicals and pesticides that add excesses estrogens and harmful chemicals. Conventional fruits and vegetables are heavily sprayed.

Ingredients – You may freeze the fruits and vegetables pieces first or buy the frozen version for a thicker smoothie.

1 Organic (if possible.) Mango
3 Organic Sweet Peaches
1 Stick if Organic Celery (including the leaf if available)
1 Small Organic Collard Green leaf
½ -1 Organic Kale leaf
A Piece of Ginger about the size of an orange seed.
Ice Cubes

Peel the mango then cut all the peaches, mango and vegetables into small pieces. Blend everything together with the ice cubes and ginger in a blender. Scoop it all out into glass cups and serve.

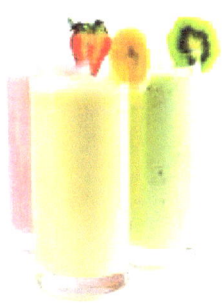

Sweet Green Vegetable and Mixed Berries Smoothie

It is healthier to use organic ingredients to avoid chemicals and pesticides that add excesses estrogens and harmful chemicals. Conventional fruits and vegetables are heavily sprayed.

Ingredients – You may freeze the fruits and vegetables pieces first or buy the frozen version for a thicker smoothie.

2 Cup of Organic Strawberries
1 Cup of Organic Blueberries
1 Cup of Organic Raspberries
1/2 Stick if Organic Celery (including the leaf if available)
1 Small Organic Collard Green leaf
½ -1 Organic Kale leaf
A Piece of Ginger about the size of an orange seed.
Ice Cubes
1 Teaspoonful of Organic Molasses - to sweeten the smoothie if necessary

Cut all the vegetables into small pieces. Blend all the berries, vegetables together with the ice cubes and ginger in a blender. Scoop it all out into glass cups and serve.

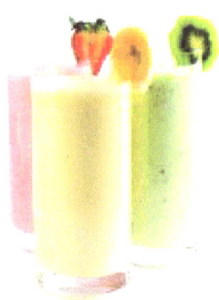

Sweet Cantaloupe Smoothie

It is healthier to use organic ingredients to avoid chemicals and pesticides that add excesses estrogens and harmful chemicals. Conventional fruits and vegetables are heavily sprayed.

Ingredients – You may freeze the Cantaloupe pieces first or buy the frozen version for a thicker smoothie.

1 Sweet Cantaloupe (Organic if possible)
½ Cup of plain Organic Yogurt (if possible get organic grass fed cow yogurt)
1 Cup of Organic skim or non-fat Milk (if possible organic grass fed milk)
Ice Cubes

Peel and cut up the cantaloupe. Blend everything together with the yogurt, milk, ice cubes and ginger in a blender. Scoop it all out into glass cups and serve.

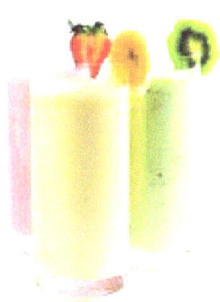

Sweet Cantaloupe and Almond Milk Smoothie

It is healthier to use organic ingredients to avoid chemicals and pesticides that add excesses estrogens and harmful chemicals. Conventional fruits and vegetables are heavily sprayed.

Ingredients – You may freeze the cantaloupe pieces first or buy the frozen version for a thicker smoothie.

1 Sweet Cantaloupe (Organic if possible)
½ Cup of Shredded Almonds (Organic if possible) you can buy the whole almonds and cut them up yourself
Plain Organic Yogurt
½ to 1 Cup of Organic Almond Milk
Ice Cubes

Peel and cut up the cantaloupe and blend everything together with the yogurt, almonds, almond milk, and ice cubes in a blender. Scoop it all out into glass cups and serve.

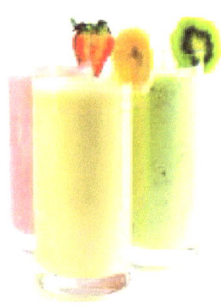

Sweet Melon and Strawberries Smoothie

It is healthier to use organic ingredients to avoid chemicals and pesticides that add excesses estrogens and harmful chemicals. Conventional fruits and vegetables are heavily sprayed.

Ingredients – You may freeze the fruits pieces first or buy the frozen version for a thicker smoothie.

2 Cups of Organic Strawberries
1 Sweet Melon (Organic if possible)
½ Cup of plain Organic Yogurt (if possible get organic grass fed cow yogurt)
1 Cup of Organic skim or non-fat Milk (if possible organic grass fed milk)
A Piece of Ginger about the size of an orange seed.
Ice Cubes

Cut up all the strawberries and the melon and blend everything together with the yogurt, milk, ice cubes and ginger in a blender. Scoop it all out into glass cups and serve.

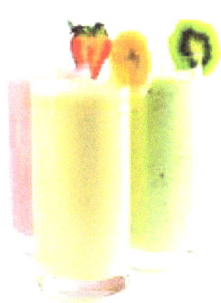

Sweet Melon and Organic Celery Smoothie

It is healthier to use organic ingredients to avoid chemicals and pesticides that add excesses estrogens and harmful chemicals. Conventional fruits and vegetables are heavily sprayed.

Ingredients – You may freeze the fruits and vegetables pieces first or buy the frozen version for a thicker smoothie.

1 Sweet Melon (Organic if possible)
1 Stick if Organic Celery (including the leaf if available)
A Piece of Ginger about the size of an orange seed.
Ice Cubes

Cut up all the strawberries and the melon and blend everything together with the yogurt, milk, ice cubes and ginger in a blender. Scoop it all out into glass cups and serve.

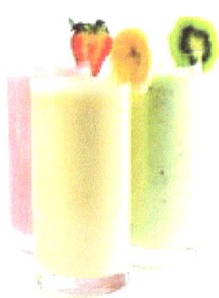

Sweet Pineapple Smoothie

It is healthier to use organic ingredients to avoid chemicals and pesticides that add excesses estrogens and harmful chemicals. Conventional fruits and vegetables are heavily sprayed.

Ingredients – You may freeze the pineapple pieces first or buy the frozen version for a thicker smoothie.

1 Sweet Pineapple
½ Cup of Shredded Almonds (Organic if possible)
1 Tablespoon of plain Organic Yogurt (if possible get organic grass fed cow yogurt)
A Piece of Ginger about the size of an orange seed.
Ice Cubes

Cut up the pineapple into small pieces. Blend everything together with the yogurt, almonds, ice cubes and ginger in a blender. Scoop it all out into glass cups and serve.

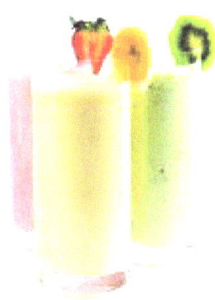

Sweet Citrus, Carrots and Green Vegetable Smoothie

It is healthier to use organic ingredients to avoid chemicals and pesticides that add excesses estrogens and harmful chemicals. Conventional fruits and vegetables are heavily sprayed.

Ingredients – You may freeze the fruits and vegetables pieces first or buy the frozen version for a thicker smoothie.

1 Organic Orange
1 Small Organic Grapefruit
1Organic Lemon
1 Mango (Organic if possible. I get mine from Shoprite)
1 Cup of Organic Carrots
1/2 Stick if Organic Celery (including the leaf if available)
1 Small Organic Collard Green leaf
½ -1 Organic Kale leaf
1 Tablespoon of plain Organic Yogurt (if possible get organic grass fed cow yogurt)
A Piece of Ginger about the size of an orange seed.
Ice Cubes

Remove only the skin from the Orange, lemon and grapefruit but leave the white peel and the seeds. The peel and seeds are very nutritional. Cut all the fruits and vegetables into small pieces. Blend everything together with the yogurt, ice cubes and ginger in a blender. Scoop it all out into glass cups and serve.

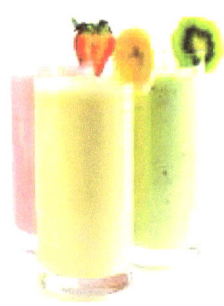

Sweet Papaya Smoothie

It is healthier to use organic ingredients to avoid chemicals and pesticides that add excesses estrogens and harmful chemicals. Conventional fruits and vegetables are heavily sprayed.

Ingredients – You may freeze the fruits and vegetables first or buy the frozen version fo a thicker smoothie.

1 Papaya
1/2 Cup of plain Organic Yogurt (if possible get organic grass fed cow yogurt)
1 Cup of plain Organic non-fat or skim Milk (if possible get organic grass fed cow milk)
1 Cup of Organic Carrots
1/2 Stick if Organic Celery (including the leaf if available)
1 Small Organic Collard Green leaf
½ -1 Organic Kale leaf
Ice Cubes

Peel and cut up the papaya into small pieces. Blend everything together with the yogurt, milk, ice cubes and in a blender. Scoop it all out into glass cups and serve.

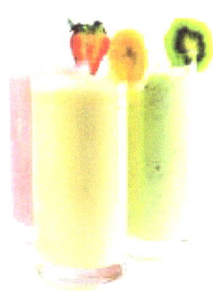

Avocado and Almond Smoothie

It is healthier to use organic ingredients to avoid chemicals and pesticides that add excesses estrogens and harmful chemicals. Conventional fruits and vegetables are heavily sprayed.

Ingredients – You may freeze the avocado pieces first or buy the frozen version for a thicker smoothie.

1 Organic Avocado
½ Cup of Shredded almonds (Organic if possible) you can buy the whole almonds and cut them up yourself
½ to 1 Cup of Organic Almond Milk
Ice Cubes

Cut up the avocado and blend everything together with the, almonds, almond milk, and ice cubes in a blender. Scoop it all out into glass cups and serve.

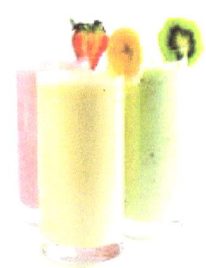

All Vegetable and Nuts Smoothie

It is healthier to use organic ingredients to avoid chemicals and pesticides that add excesses estrogens and harmful chemicals. Conventional fruits and vegetables are heavily sprayed.

Ingredients – You may freeze the vegetables pieces first or buy the frozen version for a thicker smoothie.

1 Organic Avocado
1/2 Cup of Organic Cauliflower
1 Cup of Organic Baby Carrots
1/2 Stick if Organic Celery (including the leaf if available)
1 Small Organic Collard Green leaf
½ -1 Organic Kale leaf
½ Cup of Shredded almonds (Organic if possible) you can buy the whole almonds and cut them up yourself
½ Cup of Walnuts
1 Spoonful of Organic Honey
A Piece of Ginger about the size of an orange seed.
Ice Cubes

Cut up all the vegetables and blend everything together with the, almonds, ginger, walnuts and ice cubes in a blender. Scoop it all out into glass cups and serve.

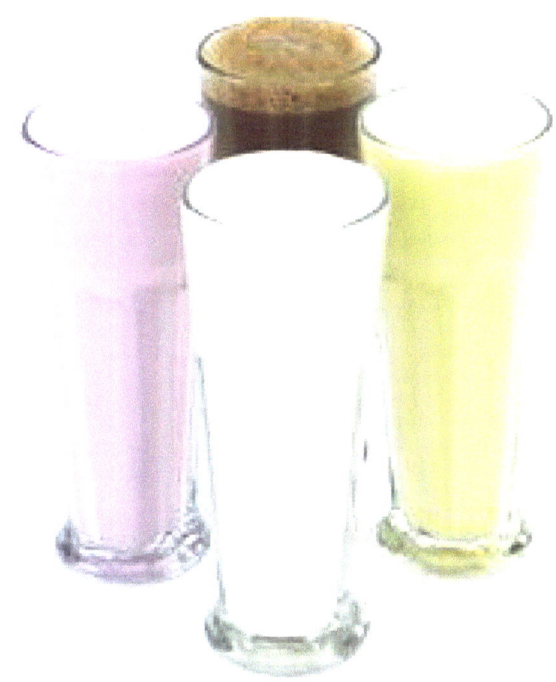

Chapter IV
Fruit, vegetable and nuts Milk Shakes

Milk Shakes are very popular. If you do not have or are unable to obtain any of the ingredients in the recipe just use what you have and substitute with other suitable ones available to you.

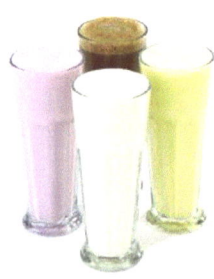

Strawberry, and Cocoa Milk Shake

It is healthier to use organic ingredients to avoid chemicals and pesticides that add excesses estrogens and harmful chemicals. Conventional fruits and vegetables are heavily sprayed.

Ingredients – You may freeze the fruits pieces first or buy the frozen version for a thicker smoothie.

1 Cup of Organic Strawberries
½ Cup of Shredded almonds (Organic if possible) you can buy the whole almonds and cut them up yourself
½ to 1 Cup of Organic Almond Milk
1 Teaspoonful of Cocoa Beans (this will give it the chocolate flavor)
Ice Cubes

Cut up the strawberries and blend everything together with the, almonds, cocoa beans, almond milk, and ice cubes in a blender. Scoop it all out into glass cups and serve.

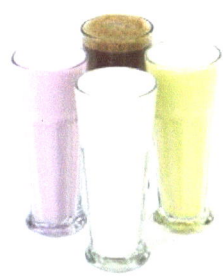

Mango, Vanilla Beans and Cantaloupe Milk Shake

It is healthier to use organic ingredients to avoid chemicals and pesticides that add excesses estrogens and harmful chemicals. Conventional fruits and vegetables are heavily sprayed.

Ingredients – You may freeze the fruits pieces first or buy the frozen version for a thicker smoothie.

1 Mango (Organic if possible)
1 Cantaloupe (Organic if possible)
1 Teaspoonful of Vanilla Essence or Ground Vanilla Beans (Organic if possible)
1 Cup of Organic Almond Milk or Goat Milk or Organic Grass fed Skim Milk or Rice Milk
Ice Cubes

Cut up the mango and cantaloupe and blend everything together with the, vanilla beans almond milk, and ice cubes in a blender. Scoop it all out into glass cups and serve.

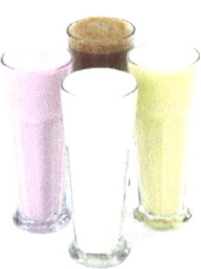

Avocado and Vanilla Beans Milk Shake

It is healthier to use organic ingredients to avoid chemicals and pesticides that add excesses estrogens and harmful chemicals. Conventional fruits and vegetables are heavily sprayed.

Ingredients – You may freeze the avocado pieces first or buy the frozen version for a thicker smoothie.

1 Avocado (Organic if possible)
1 Teaspoonful of Vanilla Essence or Ground Vanilla Beans (Organic if possible)
1 Cup of Organic Almond Milk or Goat Milk or Organic Grass fed Skim Milk or Rice Milk
Ice Cubes

Cut up the avocado and blend everything together with the, vanilla beans almond milk, and ice cubes in a blender. Scoop it all out into glass cups and serve.

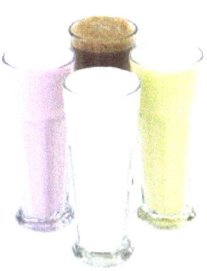

Banana and Vanilla Beans Milk Shake

It is healthier to use organic ingredients to avoid chemicals and pesticides that add excesses estrogens and harmful chemicals. Conventional fruits and vegetables are heavily sprayed.

Ingredients – You may freeze the banana pieces first or buy the frozen version for a thicker smoothie.

1 Organic Banana
1 Teaspoonful of Vanilla Essence or Ground Vanilla Beans (Organic if possible)
1 Cup of Organic Almond Milk or Goat Milk or Organic Grass fed Skim Milk or Rice Milk
Ice Cubes

Cut up the banana and blend everything together with the, vanilla beans almond milk, and ice cubes in a blender. Scoop it all out into glass cups and serve.

INDEX

A

Almond Milk, 13, 14, 21, 22, 29, 32, 35, 36, 38, 39, 40, 41
Almonds, 13, 14, 21, 22, 29, 32
Apple, 6, 9
Avocado, 35, 36, 40

B

Banana, 6, 13, 14, 16, 19, 20, 21, 24, 41
Beet, 6, 8, 22
Berries, 5, 18, 27
Blueberries, 5, 18, 27
Brown Rice, 18

C

Cantaloupe, 10, 25, 28, 29, 39
Carrots, 7, 8, 15, 17, 18, 21, 23, 33, 34, 36
Cauliflower, 4, 10, 11, 36
Celery, 4, 5, 6, 7, 8, 9, 10, 11, 16, 20, 22, 23, 24, 25, 26, 27, 31, 33, 34, 36
Citrus, 4, 5, 6, 7, 9, 13, 14, 15, 16, 17, 23, 33
Cocoa Beans, 38
Collard Green, 4, 5, 7, 8, 9, 10, 11, 22, 23, 24, 25, 26, 27, 33, 34, 36

F

Fruits, 3

G

Ginger, 4, 5, 6, 7, 8, 9, 10, 11, 15, 16, 21, 22, 23, 24, 26, 27, 30, 31, 32, 33, 36
Grapefruit, 4, 5, 6, 7, 13, 14, 15, 16, 17, 33

H

Honey, 16, 20, 25, 36

www.ingramcontent.com/pod-product-compliance
Lightning Source LLC
Chambersburg PA
CBHW041510280526
45792CB00004B/1202